TAKE 10

A Wellness Guidebook:

Wake up with More Energy
Using the 4-Step, 10-Minute Method

By
JONATHAN HODGES

Foreword by
Dr. J.J. Salehieh D.D.S.

CONTENTS

Disclaimer:
No content in this book should ever be used as a substitute for direct medical advice from your doctor or other qualified clinician.

Foreword

by Dr. J.J. Salehieh DDS

cross all medical fields, including my own—it is imperative that we operate with alertness and focus to ensure the well-being of our patients. Just like anyone else, we have families and a personal life outside of work, which is why it's vital that medical professionals also take great care of themselves. The steps outlined in this guidebook are what I have also been applying to my daily routine for years. So, I concur 100% with these steps and the benefits they provide.

This guidebook is an investment into self-care that I recommend for anyone who struggles with low energy or lack of focus. Jonathan provides a direct, yet simple methodology for how you can apply these four steps on a daily basis.

On a personal note, I've known Jonathan since he was four years old, and have always regarded him as a nice and polite young man, looking to help others. Since he joined the Air National Guard and deployed to the Middle East, I've noticed how his mindset and confidence have soared. He's now taken his willingness to help others to another level, as evidenced by writing and publishing this wellness guidebook.

With each of the four steps, he provides a basis (pillar) for why they are important. Telling someone 'what' to do is one thing, yet telling them 'why' adds more validity to the process. For example, in *Chapter 3: Focused Breathing*, he explains how vital it is to relax the mind and clear out distracting thoughts. I would also add, oftentimes if you go to sleep with worry and anxiety, you will likely wake up feeling the same way. Therefore, this step would tremendously help to push aside burdensome thoughts as you start your day.

What I also like about *TAKE 10*, is that it does not cost the user anything to implement the 4-step, 10-minute method. All it requires is your time, and what a difference those ten minutes can make! It's a simple lifestyle change that I wholeheartedly recommend.

Introduction

I thank you for taking time to read about the *4-Step, 10-Minute Method*, and I'm excited to share it with you. From the beginning, I wrote this guidebook to be as direct and concise as possible, so you can become more focused and energized each morning. I will show you how this journey began, and provide detailed information on how to apply the four steps.

The Journey...

Soon after graduating with a business degree and entering the corporate world, I noticed my stress levels rising. It wasn't just the long hours, but heavy commute traffic and physical issues related to sitting in an office all day. Hoping for change, I began extensively studying the topics of stress reduction and ergonomics. Despite this, I still dreaded waking up early. I'd hit the snooze button, eventually roll out of bed, and on my better days, stumble through an exercise routine. But I still lacked the focus and alertness I needed.

It wouldn't be until I enlisted with the Air National Guard and deployed to Kuwait that I would find the solution.

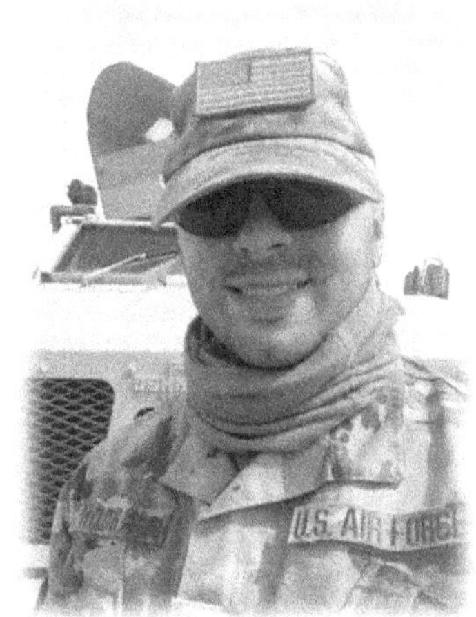

Because my deployment happened at the onset of COVID-19, strict restrictions were placed on all service members, contractors and out-of-country nationals (OCN's). As expected, we shared small living spaces and worked long hours. It was difficult to have the same level of energy we had at our home/duty stations. By April, I'd had enough. Enough of the lack of focus each morning when I got ready for work.

The desert heat, sand storms, and isolation—these were not the issue. I was the issue. Yes, I tried caffeine and everything else to "wake up" each day. A cold shower helped, yet even this wasn't enough. Then as summer arrived, there wasn't any more cold water because of the 126 degree temperature. So, over the next three months I developed a wake-to-action routine, that soon gave me a level of alertness I had never before experienced.

I'm telling you the truth: since June of 2020 I have not once needed caffeine or anything else to wake me up in the morning. When I drive onto base, I'm not yawning or craving an energy drink.

How did this happen?

It began by setting aside a little time each morning to gradually transition from being awake—to alert. I call it the *4-Step, 10-Minute Method*. It centers around the natural process of waking up both your body and mind with sleep transition. Before I discuss this process, you may have a few questions.

I drink coffee (or energy drinks) in the morning. Isn't this good enough?

I enjoy coffee and tea as much as the next guy, yet will not depend on them for energy. While caffeine and drugs have their side effects, natural remedies like focused breathing, meditation and stretching do not. In fact, just rotate the label of your 'energy' drink to see how much you know about those chemical ingredients. There is no substitute for the untapped energy and strength inside of you.

Why do I need this guidebook?

It's not uncommon to go to sleep, then wake up the next day still carrying mental burdens or anxiety—often regarding issues beyond your control. Whether you work full-time or part-time, whether you're a student or a retiree, you have a lot going on. So, if you've experienced waking up with worries and immediately focused on your busy schedule, the negative side effects can include stress, even more anxiety, and taking out internal problems onto others.

I wrote this guidebook to help reduce these negative effects. When you begin your day feeling refreshed with a positive mindset, you are likely to have more focus and energy. However, this method is not a bag of magic beans. When applied <u>regularly</u>, this method will help set you on a clearer path to supercharge your day.

How do I know your method works?

I provide various medical and wellness sources as a reference to the four steps that comprise this method. Prior to publishing, I sent copies of this book to both military members and civilians: both groups reported positive results. Some of their testimonials are also shown at the end of this book.

That said, this method (or any other one) is not guaranteed. Other inhibiting factors such as less than four hours of sleep on a regular basis, medical issues or drug use can hinder progress.

Habits are not easily broken, and you may find yourself not getting past the first step after your first attempts. Hang in there! Investing in your health is one of the best decisions you can make. Wellness is a vast topic, yet this guidebook will focus specifically on increasing your energy and focus in the morning—or whenever the time is that you begin your day.

While many have noticed an immediate change, others who tested this method found it effective after three consecutive days of application. Plus, if you only do one of these steps each morning, it is still progress that will yield a positive result!

Chapter 1: The Importance of Sleep Transition

The alarm goes off and you roll out of bed–but are you alert?

In this chapter, we will look into the transition from rest (sleep) to alertness (action).

There are plenty of sources that discuss the value of sleep, including research on the rapid eye movement (REM) cycle. Not receiving enough sleep can equate to more irritability, less focus and even a higher calorie intake.

Before I discuss each of the four steps, I'm going to describe the pillars that form the basis of this method.

Mental Focus

Yesterday's worries about friendships, relationships, money and world chaos need to be placed on hold as you wake up. How can you take good care of others, if you can't take good care of yourself first? We often burden ourselves with drama and events that are beyond our control. There will be plenty of time for you to make calls, check texts and update your calendar, so give your mind a rest.

Physical Readiness

Regardless of how many hours you sleep, your body needs a time of stillness in the morning to transition from sleep to action. You are far more complicated than a simple light switch, so don't treat yourself like one! The body needs time to adjust after spending hours motionless in sleep. Your muscular and circulatory systems need some time to transition from rest to action.

Independence from Chemical Dependence

Yes, coffee and tea are great—but we should not depend on them for energy. Instead, keep a glass of water on your nightstand so you can rehydrate after waking up.

You're in Control

I believe that even small investments into your health will yield greater returns over time. Walking outside, eating responsibly, practicing good hygiene–it just takes one step at a time. At the end of the day, *you* control the direction of your health. Will you go backward, or forward? In the following chapters, we will discuss disengagement, focused breathing, meditation and light stretching.

Chapter 2: Ignore All Distraction

Who loves being dragged from a comfortable sleep by a noisy alarm? Wouldn't it be nice to sleep in whenever you wanted, on your own schedule? Perhaps in heaven, but on earth even billionaire CEO's need to keep up with demanding schedules. As a result, it's important that when you wake up—you allow your mind to relax and not burden it with any distraction.

Benefits: your mental focus will be stronger if external content is not overwhelming you.

Choose a Good Alarm

Try switching to a subtle alarm sound, whether it's ocean waves or chirping birds. Sudden sounds are unpleasant and do not place you in a good mood. If you own one of those buzzer alarms that send off a static noise, please pick it up—and gently toss it into a garbage bin. There are far better options, such as the scheduled bedtime feature on your smartphone, or a light alarm clock that slowly lightens up the room.

This first step is difficult, yet doable. It may take you a while. To clear away distractions, <u>begin with the following:</u>

- Stop your alarm and do not press snooze.

- Do not check social media, status updates, or work emails.

Position Yourself

- Sit up on the edge of your bed, or go into another room and sit upright in a chair (not a couch or recliner).

- Bring your phone/timer with you.

Keep in Mind...

Your status updates and social media likes will still be there later in the day. This moment is for you. Next, we will combine this with mental preparation as you awaken.

Chapter 3: Focused Breathing

Focused breathing will help prepare and relax the mind each morning. Whether you slept comfortably or not, this three-minute breathing exercise will help propel you to a stage of alertness and focus. Focused breathing can also be referred to as chest and diaphragmatic breathing.

Benefits: focused breathing can help lower blood pressure and reduce stress.

This 2nd step will last for three minutes.

Just as your body is given time to relax, so should your mind. The following guide is intended to help you clear your mind of pesky thoughts.

The Four Stages of Focused Breathing:

1. While sitting upright, place your left hand on your stomach and your right hand on your chest

2. As you inhale through the nose and exhale out the mouth, breathe **ten times** into your chest. As you breathe, your chest will both press into *and* pull away from your right hand. Try to keep your stomach area still, as it is your chest that's receiving most of the oxygen intake.

3. Next, breathe into the lower lungs **ten times**. With every inhale, your stomach will both press into and pull away from your left hand. The goal is for oxygen to reach the lower portion of your lungs, which often requires deeper breaths.

4. Now take **ten full breaths**. You will do this by breathing into both your stomach and chest at the same time. Remember: there are <u>no</u> worries or tasks on your mind. This is a moment to relax and reset. Focus on your breathing.

Posture

Try to keep your shoulders as level as possible, so that when you inhale you are not lifting up with your shoulders. Practice this style of breathing throughout the day (responsibly). In other words, do not close your eyes and breathe deeply while driving a car, train or commercial aircraft.

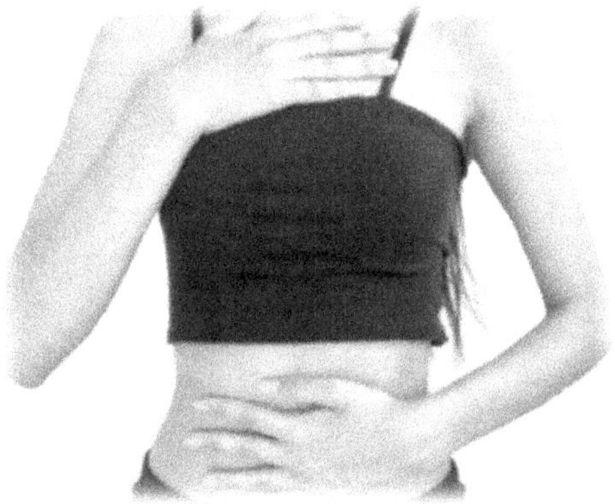

The next step will further improve your mental focus.

Chapter 4: Meditation

You've heard of meditation, but have you ever practiced it? This step will help guide you into a much clearer focus as you begin the day. But before you ease out of bed, remember to keep your mind <u>free of worry</u>. There is only so much you can do, and this time is for you to gradually transition into a new level of focus and energy.

Background

The topic of meditation is a broad one because it varies by style and culture. For many people it is part of their daily routine, whether practiced for three minutes or thirty minutes. Here I will describe it from a general (introductory) point of view.

Benefits: Meditation can help reduce stress and promote relaxation.

Being spiritually minded, I can also attest to the value of prayer. Oftentimes, I find that prayer in solitude can relieve my worries and take me to a greater place. Maybe it does for you as well.

This 3rd step will last for three minutes.

The goal is to put yourself at ease and detach from events that are beyond your control. Remember, your tasks and schedules can wait. This time is for you.

How to Begin:

- ○ Sit comfortably in a quiet place.

- ○ Close your eyes.

- ○ Your mind will soon shift to <u>only</u> positive and peaceful thoughts.

- ○ Continue to take deep and consistent breaths.

- ○ Think about what you are grateful for.

- ○ Focus on the good that you can accomplish.

- ○ Your worries and mistakes are behind you, only opportunities are in front of you.

Stay Positive

Dwelling on negativity or challenges will only raise your stress levels and defeat the purpose of this exercise. During this step, try to also maintain a small smile. This can help produce a more positive attitude by releasing endorphins and serotonin. By the way, rumor has it that forty-three muscles are required to frown, and only seventeen needed to smile.

The next step is physical: waking up the body.

Chapter 5: Light Stretching

When you get ready for the day and leave your residence, it's important that you are physically refreshed.

Why Stretching?

Your muscular and circulatory systems have been at rest while you sleep. This final step will help energize as you transition from rest to action. You've probably seen athletes and fitness experts stretch prior to a game or exercise; yet in this case I will discuss it on a smaller scale.

Benefits: Light stretching can help increase your flexibility and improve posture. There are many stretching options available, depending on your flexibility and experience level.

Target Areas

Here I provide five effective stretches that target your hip, groin, abdomen, IT band, as well as your upper and lower back. Please feel free to try other ones if you prefer. If you do not own a yoga mat, please buy one after reading this guidebook.

- Seated Groin Stretch

- Hip Opener and Groin Stretch

- Seated Stretch

- Prone Press-up Stretch

- Lateral Side Stretch

Please Remember...

As you rotate between these, do no more than 30 consecutive seconds for each stretch. If you want to do a certain stretch for one minute, just divide it into smaller increments. If you are currently injured or under a doctor's orders, please avoid the stretching portion altogether until you feel safe to proceed.

Observable Improvements

As stretching continues to be part of your daily routine, you may notice improvements to your posture. For optimal benefits, consider doing this throughout the day. Even if you're at work, take a few short breaks to periodically stretch, even if it's for 15-30 seconds.

Instruction:

1) Sit flat on the ground with your back and head positioned straight up.

2) Now spread your knees and touch the soles of your feet together, and stabilize with both of your hands.

3) Gently lean forward and hold for about 10 seconds. Then lean back to a neutral position to rest for 10 seconds.

Muscles being stretched:
Adductor longis, adductor magnus, pectineus, gracilis, lower latissimus dorsi, pectineus, middle sartorius

Seated Groin Stretch

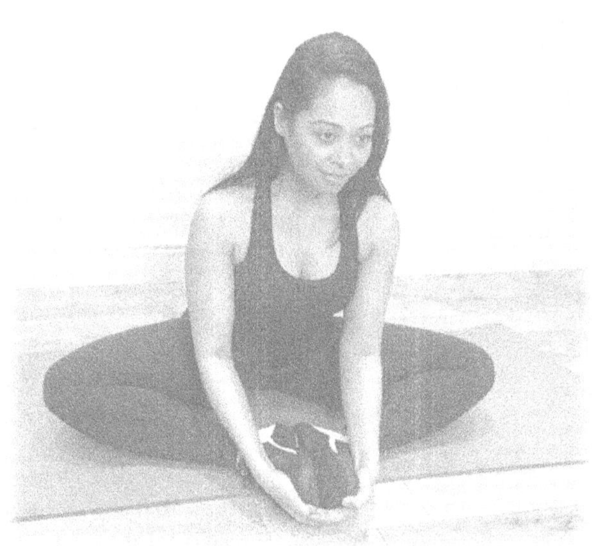

Hip Opener and Groin Stretch

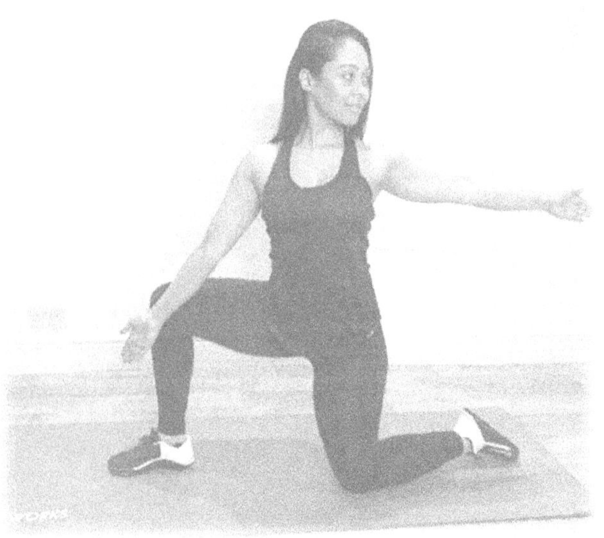

Instruction:

1) Plant your right foot forward on the ground, and kneel with the left leg also positioned forward.

2) Your left heel will face upward and toes touch the ground.

3) Stabilize your right wrist against the inner knee that is planted, and slowly twist your torso to the left. Use your free arm to stretch outward as you twist.

4) Turn your head and neck along with your torso. Then hold for 15-20 seconds; next, switch sides and repeat.

Muscles being stretched:
Adductor magnus, gracilis, middle sartorius

<u>Seated Stretch</u>

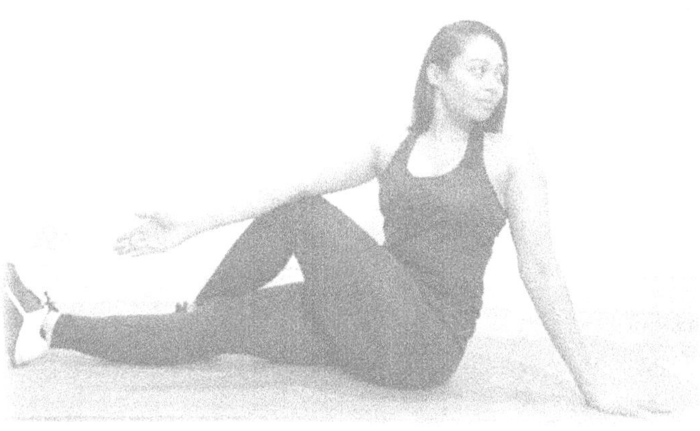

Muscles being stretched: gluteus medius, lower latissimus dorsi, gluteus maximus

Instruction:

1) Sit flat on the ground, place your left leg over the right leg, and set your left hand flat on the ground to stabilize.

2) Slowly pull your bent knee towards your chest, using your extended elbow to stabilize your crossed knee.

3) Gently twist your upper body as if to look over your left shoulder.

4) Hold for at least 15 seconds, and then switch legs to work the other side.

<u>Prone Press-up Stretch</u>

Instruction:

1) Lie face down (prone) on the floor.

2) Place your palms flat, with fingertips facing forward—positioned alongside your chest.

3) Slowly arch your back upwards, keeping your thighs on the ground. Continue to maintain this arch for at least 15 seconds, and slowly breathe. Then come back down to briefly rest before repeating.

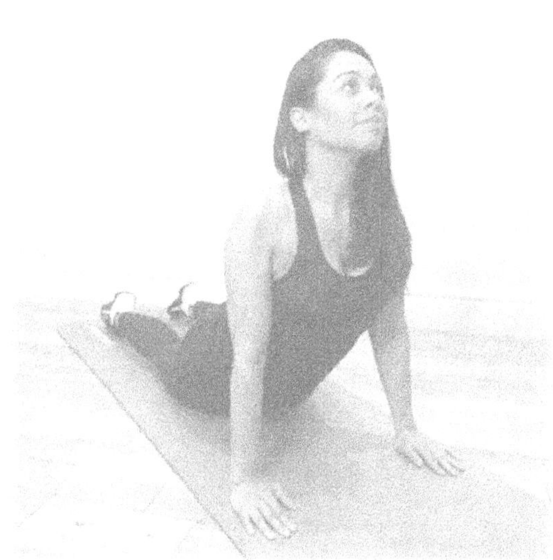

Muscles being stretched:
External oblique, internal oblique, rectus abdominis

<u>Lateral Side Stretch</u> *(3 poses)*

Instruction:

1) Stand straight up, and extend both arms over your head.

2) Take hold of your left wrist with the right hand. Gently lean towards the left and hold for 5 seconds. *Try not to arch your back forward or backward, only tilt to the side.*

3) Align back to the center.

4) Now stretch to the right, and hold for 5 seconds.

5) Align back to center.

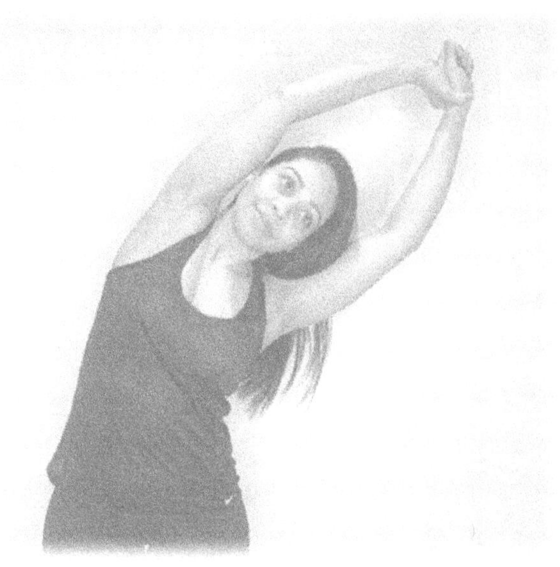

Muscles being stretched:
Serratus anterior, latissimus dorsi, external oblique, iliacus

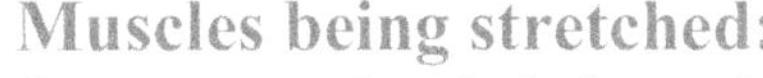

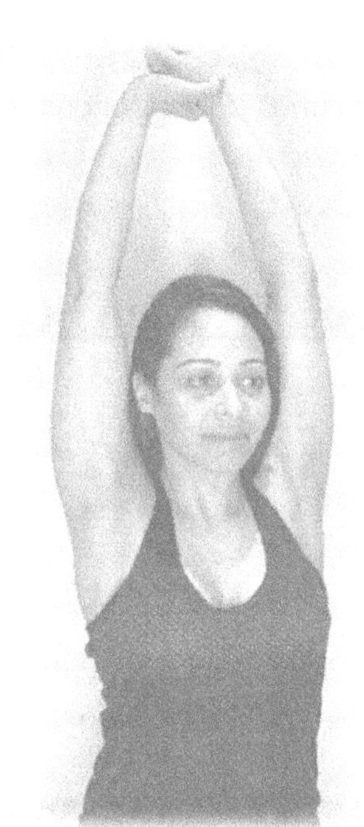

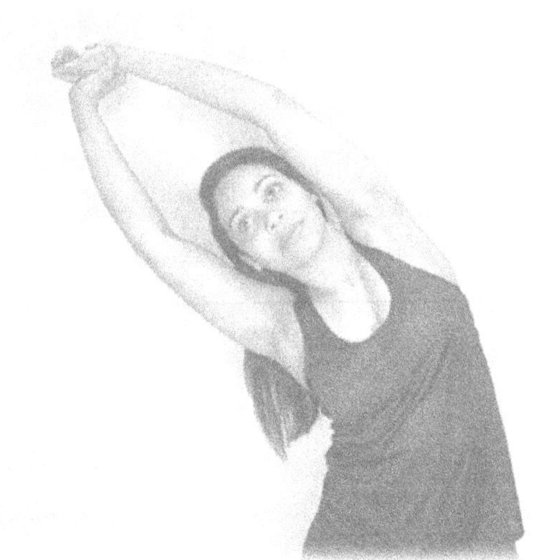

Chapter 6: Your Wellness Journey

Oftentimes, our physical problems are self-inflicted through a number of active and passive behaviors that constantly produce negativity. I'm going to explain what these are, and how you can remedy this. Keep in mind, the 4-step method is just one example of how you can invest a small amount of time each day to produce a positive outcome.

Active behaviors are ones you are fully aware of. If you smoke cigarettes every day and eat or drink large quantities of processed sugar, these are damaging <u>active</u> behaviors. You willingly accept the outcome and problems these actions produce.

Passive behaviors are actions you take that are habitual or unintentional. If you sit for extended periods of time leaning forward at a desk, eventually you will develop an unhealthy posture. If you use a basic computer mouse, twisting your wrist, you may develop Carpal Tunnel Syndrome over the years.

As part of your wellness journey, please take more time to assess what habits and actions that you need to improve—or completely remove. There are people who look up to and care about you, so your decisions do not impact just yourself. The decades will pass us by, and with age comes physical challenges that we will either conquer, or be conquered by. You have what it takes to go beyond where you are right now!

Conclusion

Thank you for taking the time to read this Guidebook.

This was time well spent as an investment into your health. Going forward, if you have difficulty following through with this method after a few attempts, then no problem...keep on trying! Over time you may find yourself adding to this method, and ten minutes will just be a starting point. Remember, whether you walk or run on your wellness journey—keep moving forward, never backward.

Contact Info:

I enjoy hearing success stories from satisfied readers. Reach out and share yours at **take10foryou@gmail.com**. I'm available to answer any questions you may have about the 4-step method. Please also stay tuned for the audiobook version of this guidebook.

Notes

Page 6
Source Camille, Peri. 10 Things to Hate About Sleep Loss. WebMD: Sleep Disorders. February 13, 2014. Accessed March. 17, 2021. https://www.webmd.com/sleep-disorders/features/10-results-sleep-loss

Page 9
Source Peterson, Laura A. R.N. *Decrease Stress By Using Your Breath*. MAYO Clinic: Stress Management. March 23, 2017. Accessed Feb. 15, 2021. https://www.mayoclinic.org/healthy-lifestyle/stress-management/in-depth/decrease-stress-by-using-your-breath/art-20267197

Page 9
Source Bullock, B Grace. PhD. How to Fight Stress with Intentional Breathing. Mindful.Org. Feb. 6, 2017. Accessed Feb. 10, 2021. https://www.mindful.org/fight-stress-intentional-breathing/

Page 9
Source Bullock, B Grace. PhD. What Focusing on the Breath Does to Your Brain. Greater Good Science Journal. October 31, 2019. Accessed Jan. 19, 2021. https://greatergood.berkeley.edu/article/item/what_focusing_on_the_breath_does_to_your_brain.

Page 10
Source Harvard Health Publishing. Relaxation techniques: Breath control helps quell errant stress response. July 6, 2020. Accessed Jan. 14, 2021. https://www.health.harvard.edu/mind-and-mood/relaxation-techiques-breath-control-helps-quell-errant-stress-response

Page 10
Source Stibich, Mark PhD. Top 10 Reasons You Should Smile Every Day. February 19, 2021. Accessed March 10, 2021. https://www.verywellmind.com/top-reasons-to-smile-every-day-2223755

Page 10
Source Abee, Blair. The Meditation Book. 2017. Vallejo, CA. 2nd Edition, Energetic Wave Publishing

Page 10
Source National Center for Complementary and Integrative Health. Meditation: In Depth. April, 2016. Accessed Jan. 6, 2021. https://www.nccih.nih.gov/health/meditation-in-depth

Page 10
Source Harvard Health Publishing. How meditation helps with depression. February 12, 2021. Accessed Feb. 18, 2021. https://www.health.harvard.edu/mind-and-mood/how-meditation-helps-with-depression

Pages 11-13
Source Nelson, Arnold G., Kokkonen, Jouko. (2014) Stretching Anatomy, Second Edition. Champaign, IL. Human Kinetics Publishing

Acknowledgements

To my military co-workers, thank you for being the first to successfully test this routine.

To writer Johanna Hickle, thank you for your talented proofreading skills.

User Reviews

This works. While it took me a few days to notice a change, one effect is that I am more eager to go about every day activities. The key—is consistency. I've been trying this method for the last few weeks, and want to make it a habit.

J. Lor
Merced, CA

Even though I go to the gym each morning, the other three steps are extremely helpful, especially the one about disengaging from my phone
right after waking up.

S. Valentina
Phoenix, AZ

The 4-step 10-minute method is a quick and easy way to begin my day. The breathing and meditation steps really do make a difference. Simple techniques, yet a huge difference.

G. Simpson
Vacaville, CA

A morning routine is an investment. It shows that an investment is made on the most important person—yourself! Jonathan has written an elegantly simple and practical guide on how to best start your day, and it only takes 10 minutes!

K. Bagatsing
Redwood City, CA

Reading this book has given me pause about my daily routines. For instance, completely giving up energy drinks is not something I'm ready to do, however my intake has decreased since applying this method over the last few months.

R. Lance
Houston, TX

I've practiced meditation for years, and agree 100% with the steps outlined in this book. However, I didn't have much of an exercise routine, and the stretching portion has been a great starting point for me.

V. Naylor
Salt Lake City, UT

Pages intentionally left blank